YOGA, I Become……

A Simple Yoga Guide for Everyone, to Become Healthy in Mind, Body and Soul and also a Yoga Devotee.

Table of Contents

Other books by this Publisher *Awere First Publishing:-*

- GO TO our website: www.awerefirstpublishing.com OR check on ourlist:

- ALSO, you can follow us on our various *Social Media Platforms:-*

    o **PINTEREST**: kindlebooks8566

    o **YouTube**: AwereFirstPublishing CHANNEL

    o **LINKEDIN**: linkedin.com/in/awerefirst-publishing-26870417b

    o **TWITTER**: https://twitter.com/Awerefirstpubl1

    o (Audiobook_samples)**SOUNDCLOUD**: www.soundcloud.com/awerefirstpublishing

- Other books by **R. ESPIRITO** :-

    o EMPATHY: A 10-STEP GUIDE TO EMPATHY, EMPATHY AND YOU..... OR (https://amzn.to/2uNRqu4)

Introduction

I want to thank you and congratulate you for downloading this book, '*YOGA, I Become - A Simple Yoga Guide for Everyone, to Become Healthy in Mind, Body and Soul and also a Yoga Devotee.*'

How stressed are you? Do you feel that no matter what you do, you just can't seem to find the sense of peace you are looking for? Do you long for holidays assuming that drifting off to a faraway island or going on an expensive vacation can offer you the peace you are craving? No, I am not against you taking vacations. And sure, a holiday can be rejuvenating for a short period of time, but as soon as the good feelings wear off, you are back to facing the daily stresses of life. What do you do then? You can't wait another 6 months so that you can get your dose of bliss, can you?

If you are looking for a permanent solution, a life that doesn't constantly need you to get away from your daily life, take my advice and join a yoga class right away. If you are a beginner and wish to know everything about yoga, its different forms, techniques, poses and stretches, you have stumbled upon the perfect guide. I hope you will enjoy reading this book and start your yoga journey soon. Happy reading!!

Thanks again for downloading this book, I hope you enjoy it!

Chapter 1: What is Yoga?

Yoga is defined as the science of self-realization. For some, it also means a union of the spirit, body and the mind. Yoga is a science as well as an art. This ancient science that finds its roots in India is now practiced by people across the globe. In the following chapters you will learn more about yoga.

You may have decided to take up yoga – but after looking for yoga classes in your vicinity, your head is spinning. Which form of yoga should you take up? The Vinyasa or hot yoga? And for those of you who have no clue what either one of these are, I am talking about the different forms of yoga.

If you are a newbie, you may want to educate yourself about these yoga techniques and then decide which one is best for you. Some of these techniques are mentioned below:

Hatha Yoga

Hatha yoga is a slow moving yoga practice that requires you to hold a specific pose for a few breaths. As a beginner, you may find it somewhat boring or difficult to stay in the same pose for more than 5 seconds, but that's fine. As you continue to practice these poses, you will start enjoying the process. A lot of yoga studios teach this gentler form of yoga, but if you can't find the right classes, you can even learn the basics from yoga videos on YouTube.

The term "hatha" is Sanskrit for any kind of yoga practice that teaches physical postures. It's basically a practice of the body, which balances out two different energies.

Vinyasa yoga

You can quickly get in flow using this dynamic yoga practice that connects breath and movement together in an almost dance-like way. This is especially fun for those of you who find it boring to perform the slow yoga forms. In most Vinyasa yoga sessions, you won't be required to linger long in every single pose; the pace can be quicker than other yoga forms, so get ready for your heart-rate to rise. A lot of yoga teachers will play music and have their students match the beat to the sequence of the yoga poses.

Got high intensity work out lovers, this form of yoga can offer you the rush you experience after an intense workout session because of its faster pace. Most endurance athletes, as well as runners, are attracted to the vinyasa yoga because of the rapid and continuous movement.

Iyengar yoga

This form of yoga might require you to pay extra attention to your body's alignment in every single pose. You will soon become friends with props such as straps, blankets or even a ropes wall. All these props are aimed at helping you perform within a range of motion, which is not only safe, but also effective. Each posture in the Iyengar yoga is held for an extended period of time. Don't let this overwhelm you though; you can always start slow and then take it a few notches up. If you are new to yoga, then it's wiser to start with a level one of Iyengar yoga to help you familiarize with this particular technique.

This form of yoga, although meant for detail-oriented yogis, can be immensely beneficial for everyone. Moreover, the Iyengar yoga can be practiced by people of all ages and is also great for those who are suffering from injuries. It's advisable to consult your doctor before you go ahead with this yoga form.

Ashtanga yoga

If you are looking to challenge yourself a bit, you should certainly try out Ashtanga yoga. This form of yoga consists of six different series of specifically created yoga poses to help you breathe through each pose properly. You will breathe and flow through every yoga pose with an aim to build internal heat. However, there's a catch. You will be performing the same poses in the same manner in every single class. It is advisable to perform this form of yoga under strict supervision, as the poses are slightly tricky. Follow your instructor and do not perform any pose without getting the form correct.

Bikram yoga

Do you love the rush you experience when you break a sweat? Well, then get ready for Bikram yoga. Bikram yoga involves a series of 26 different yoga poses including two breathing exercises that are practiced in a heated room with approximately 40 percent humidity. All the studios that teach Bikram yoga follow the same sequence for each pose, so you will know exactly what you need to do once you unroll your mat. Again, if you are new to yoga, you need to take it easy without letting the process get to you. Rest and hydrate well before you attend the Bikram yoga sessions. This type of yoga is ideal for people who like to follow a particular routine.

Hot yoga

This form of yoga is as hot as it sounds, I mean literally. Hot yoga is practiced in a heated room and is somewhat similar to Bikram yoga. The only difference is that the teachers or the students aren't constrained by the 26-pose sequence of Bikram yoga. The heat in the room can make you move much closer to your body as compared to the non-heated class, but you have to ensure to not overstretch yourself or push beyond your actual capacity. You may be excited about this yoga, as it is very calming, but proceed with caution.

If you are a sweat-lover, you will enjoy this hard-core workout that will leave you drenched.

Kundalini yoga

Several Hollywood celebrities such as author Gabrielle Bernstein and actor Russell Brand have popularized this form of yoga. This is a particularly mentally and physically challenging practice that appears different from your normal yoga class. Here, you will be performing repetitive physical exercises along with some intense breath work while singing, chanting and meditating. What's the goal of this yoga form? To break through the internal barriers of your mind and body while allowing the untapped energy residing inside of you to release. This helps to bring a greater level of self-awareness.

This form of yoga is ideal for people who are attracted to spiritual practices in general. People who are seeking something beyond a mere workout may end up enjoying Kundalini owing to its emphasis on meditation, breath work and spiritual energy.

Restorative yoga

A lot of you may feel like you are not doing a lot in a restorative yoga session... but that's the whole point. This form of yoga involves a slow moving and a rather mellow practice with longer holds which allow your body a chance for tapping into the parasympathetic nervous system. This, in turn, allows a person to experience deeper relaxation. Here, you will be using props such as bolsters, blankets and even yoga blocks for supporting your entire body through every single pose.

It's best for just about anyone and everyone. This yoga practice is ideal for people who struggle with slowing down, or anxiety or someone who has experienced insomnia for an extended period of time. It is also greatly beneficial for athletes on their recovery days.

Yin Yoga

If you wish to find a sense of calm and a mind and body balance, there's no better way than yoga. Yin Yoga, which is completely opposite to a faster-paced Ashtanga, requires you to hold the poses for several minutes at a time. This particular practice is created for targeting your deeper connective tissues while restoring your body's elasticity as well as muscle strength. You may feel a tiny bit antsy at first when you start practicing this form of yoga, but if you hand around for a few classes, you might find yourself hooked to its restorative powers.

It's best for people who have a constant need to unwind and stretch, especially individuals whose work involves sitting behind a desk for longer hours. That said, Yin yoga is not advised for people who are too flexible as you might end up overdoing a few poses.

Chapter 2: The Five Principles of Yoga

There are five basic principles that underpin every form of yoga. These will allow you a starting point for understanding this mystically and sometimes-vast school of thought.

Beneficial exercise

Sometimes, yoga is looked upon incorrectly as an undemanding form of physical activity. But the truth is that yoga routines can offer you the benefit of a complete cardio workout while increasing your aerobic stamina.

When you practice yoga sequences that are often strenuous, you will feel the same rush you feel after an intense workout. So, if you are someone who is quick to write off yoga as a non-challenging form of exercise, think again. Yoga offers various poses that bring about a perfect balance between your body and mind. Through yoga, you can also stretch and massage your internal organs, tone the muscles as well as ligaments, improve blood circulation in all parts of the body and joints and also enhance the flexibility of your spine. Regardless of whichever exercise regime you wish to follow, your overall fitness, stamina and medical conditions should be taken into consideration. When it comes to yoga, your postures can be modified using different aids for ensuring a safe, but effective practice for everyone.

Correct breathing

We often don't realize this, but most of us breathe incorrectly. Yoga places a great emphasis on your breath and considers it a bridge between your physical body and the mind. When you breathe correctly, you take full and rhythmic breaths, employing the lung capacity for maximizing the intake of oxygen. To achieve deep breathing that is full, rhythmical and slow, you need to regulate the duration and depth of inhalation as well as exhalation.

Yoga breathing techniques can leave you feeling completely rejuvenated by maximizing the oxygen levels in your blood. Precise execution of the postures is required for ensuring that you breathe correctly throughout the exercise session. When you adopt the poses, you need to be extra aware of your upper torso while allowing your ribs to be lifted up, chest to be open, and a connection to the movements of your diaphragm. Taking deep breaths also helps to eliminate the stale air stored in your lungs. It also increases your energy levels as you take control of your breath, thereby helping you to accomplish a much focused and calmer mind.

Complete relaxation

Yoga defines a complete state of true freedom from the stresses of the world. It's a true form of relaxation as it encourages the body to consume minimum amount of energy that is required for existence. Yoga distinguishes between the mental, physical and even the spiritual relaxation of a person, allowing each of these factors to be accomplished in different ways. For instance, physical relaxation requires you to use movements to loosen and disperse the areas of tension in your body, which are a result of trapped negative energies. Relaxation sequences focus on increasing your capacity to feel the tension in all these areas and then apply gentle pressure on them in order to release tension. This can also be similar to the techniques used in acupressure.

Balanced diet

If you follow yoga, you can't be eating truckloads of junk and expect to get the results. Yoga requires you to mindful of whatever you put in your mouth. NO more stuffing your face with cookies and pizza. The yogic approach to a healthy diet is much similar to the modern ideas of healthy eating. So, if you are a healthy eater already, you might not struggle with following the yogic diet. Yoga teachings promote consuming a lot of fresh fruit, vegetables, pulses, nuts and dairy. A lot of importance is placed on the way we eat these foods rather than just paying attention to what we are eating. Switching off the television or keeping away from your mobile phone helps you get mindful about the food you are consuming. You are also required to eat at a slightly slower pace than you generally do. This helps to encourage the body's ability to ingest, digest, and absorb nutrients present in the food.

The general rules of yogic eating are to always eat in moderation, eating only when hungry, chewing your food properly at your own pace, eating at specific times of the day, minimizing your fluid intake during the meals and a positive approach towards what you are consuming as well as the food preparation.

Positive thinking

We all know the magic of positive thinking, and we also know that we cannot think positively all the time. Yoga helps to redirect our negative thoughts whenever they occur towards the positive aspects of our lives. It places a huge importance for sustaining your mental wellbeing. Yoga uses relaxation and meditation techniques for consciously clearing our minds off all the negative energies we tend to take on. It also helps us in employing various types of positive affirmations to increase our self-esteem.

When you are easily able to put aside your negative thinking and emotions, you will start identifying your strengths and weaknesses in a realistic fashion. Now, to reverse the negative wiring of your brain may take some time, as it's not easy to shed a massive momentum of the mind. But when you start practicing yoga regularly, you automatically follow a self-discipline that eventually brings you closer to a state of serenity and harmony.

Chapter 3: Benefits of Yoga

Is there anything yoga cannot offer? Right from stress relief to reduction in blood pressure to weight loss, it offers numerous benefits to people. And it's not a bad practice either. In fact, yoga has been in existence since…

Although there are countless benefits of yoga, we have narrowed down the list to 10 of the most important benefits it has to offer.

Improvement in flexibility

Let's start with the most talked about and the most obvious benefit of practicing regular yoga. Yoga poses are basically designed to increase the strength and stretch ability of the muscles, thereby making them flexible. Flexibility is a natural by-product of stretching your body in different ways while controlling your breath. That said; do not confuse stretching exercises with yoga. Yoga is much more than that. Once the flexibility in your muscles increase, it results in better blood circulation, healing of pains and aches, increased balance and improvement in posture among other benefits.

So, whether your goal is to perform the perfect splits or not, your body is sure going to be extra flexible. Practicing yoga for 2-3 times in a week can significantly improve your flexibility. When you are super flexible, you also lower your chances of injuries and drop in energy levels.

Improves posture

Do you walk with a hump? Do you have droopy shoulders? Does your posture signal low confidence? I have a solution for you. If you perform any of these yoga poses including mountain pose, tree pose, cat cow pose, the standing forward fold, downward facing dog, cobra pose, bow pose, or warrior I, you can improve your posture to a great extent. In fact, we all could use some posture training for our bodies. Amidst this busy life, we often forget to pay attention to our postures especially when we are sitting in the chair working all day, or doing household chores. Incorrect posture cannot only convey low confidence, but it can also put pressure on your joints.

Most of us underestimate the importance of having a good posture, but it's key to maintaining a well-balanced life. A good posture can ensure that your muscles, joints and bones are in proper alignment with each other. This can in-turn increases your efficiency. A good posture speaks volumes about your personality as a whole. It impacts your almost every system in the body including, muscular, digestive, and nervous and the circulatory system. Practicing yoga regularly can not only enhance your posture, but also ensure that your body is in perfect functioning condition.

Relieves aches and pains

This is especially helpful if you are an athlete, someone who loves to work out on a regular basis, or spends long hours at work. Aches and pains are caused by various factors including internal as well as external. Regardless of whether your pain is temporary or permanent, yoga can always give you relief.

Several researchers from Duke University Medical Centre studies the effects of yoga on humans and concluded that one of the health benefits yoga offers is that treats chronic pain which can be caused by various afflictions, which includes carpal tunnel syndrome, osteoarthritis and even fibromyalgia.

The researchers also concluded that the participants in these studies not only experience a relief form stiff joints and muscles but also experienced an increase in their muscle strength as well as flexibility.

Exercises like distance running and weightlifting puts extra pressure and strain on our muscles that can weaken them after a due course of time. Even if you are runner or love performing intense exercises, you can practice yoga as an alternative activity, which will help soothe and even cure inflamed joints. Pills can certainly come in handy for relieving pain, but there's nothing like a flexibility exercise like yoga, which not only relieves pains and aches but also doesn't cause any side effect.

Helps in weight loss

Most people think that yoga is only about breathing right, meditating and stretching your muscles. While this belief is true, what they don't know is that yoga can also help them lose weight over a period of time. The weight loss that occurs as a result of practicing regular yoga can sustain for a long time. Unlike other weight loss techniques where the weight loss can come back with a vengeance once you stop following them, with yoga, there are less to no chances of gaining weight again. It is an incredibly powerful tool which, when applied correctly can give you dramatic weight loss results.

Yoga has also been proven to lower your cortisol levels. Cortisol is a stress hormone, which causes belly fat and results in weight gain. A lot of people think that they have to work out for hours in the gym or run miles before they can see any weight loss results, it couldn't be further from truth. IN fact, long distance running can raise your cortisol levels, thereby causing stress and resulting in weight gain.

If your goal is weight loss, and you don't wish to go through grueling forms of exercise, then you should definitely consider yoga. Regularly practicing yoga can help burn fat, build muscle and burn calories from your body.

Relieves stress and anxiety

Stress is a part of our daily lives. There's no way we can avoid stress from our lives completely, but we can certainly manage stress while keeping our mind and body feeling lighter. This is also another benefit of yoga that a lot of people are unaware of. Yoga can actually help relieve stress and anxiety from your lives, making you a much healthier and resilient person. People are so busy these days shuffling between their family and work life, that they are left with no time to unwind. We have less privacy, less time and more stress than ever.

We don't realize it often, but stress and anxiety can cause a major damage to your body if left untreated. As mentioned earlier, this very stress causes our bodies to release a hormone caused cortisol which leads to weight gain and a whole lot of other problems. Typically, meditation is suggested as a remedy for lowering stress. But regardless of whether you decide to include meditation during your yoga practice or not, simply performing some yoga poses can lower your anxiety and stress levels to a great extent.

Builds muscle

The worst part about aging is that people start to lose muscle, making them appear older and low on energy. Practicing a relaxing yoga poses repeatedly can actually help build your body's muscle strength. Yes, as unbelievable as it sounds, it is actually possible to build muscle without lifting any weight.

Yoga is all about slow movements and controlled poses that aim at strengthening your muscles and making your joints more flexible among other things. Most yoga poses require you to hold or lift a specific portion of your body up in the air. Although this may seem impossible at the start with some discipline, you can certainly nail these poses. This does require a lot of strength, and yoga helps you build that power. Yoga is basically made of bodyweight exercises that will gradually help you to build muscle if you continue to improve your practice and challenge yourself.

Enhances your sleep pattern

Just like insomnia is a common problem among people who are stressed, or anxious, some may even suffer from excessive sleep patterns. Not all of us react to stress in the same way. While most of us find it difficult to sleep when we are stressed, some of us sleep for excessively long hours as a way of fighting stress. Both these sleep patterns are inherently faulty and can cause serious damage to your nervous system, body and mind as a whole.

You cannot underestimate the power of a good night's sleep. Sleep can help the body recover from the stress we experience each day. Its no wonder that we are often recommended by the doctor to get at least 8 hours sleep every day. This is how our bodies heal. On the other hand, if you find yourself difficult to stay awake, this can also pose as a health risk. Fortunately, yoga can cure both the problems.

Here are some tips for you to sleep better:

- Eliminate distractions (minimize the use of cell phone, laptop or even TV)
- Ensure that the temperature of your bedroom is warm enough.
- Use blackout curtains to ensure that the room is dark enough while you sleep.

Following these tips along with regular yoga practice can ensure a better sleep pattern, thereby improving your overall health.

Improves balance

A lot of people are naturally gifted with perfect balance. While others like me feel like having "butterfingers" most of the time as we go along dropping and picking things. You see, balance and stability are also an important factor that has been highly underrated. As we start aging, we may start losing our mobility skills. While this does not happen with everyone, this is what a lot of people experience. A lot of people may be eons away from experiencing something like this and Kudos to you for staying fit in spite of your age.

Now, the rest of us might need some help when it comes to our balancing skills. This is where yoga comes in the picture. No matter how old you are, almost everyone can perform yoga poses to enhance their stability and balance. Yoga can't help someone build balance, stability and strength, but it can also change your self-perception. Your self-perception can change the way you look at yourself and help increase your self-esteem. When you start looking at yourself in a positive light, you raise your value as a person, helping you easily achieve success in whichever field you desire.

Releases tension

Do you feel tension in your muscles especially when you are going through an episode of anxiety and stress? Chances are that all the stiffness and tension that had built up in your bodies is affecting your shoulders and neck area. This is one reason why you feel incredibly good when someone gives you a shoulder or a neck massage.

Our muscles can stiffen up as we age, thanks to our sedentary lifestyles. Sitting behind a computer screen or in front of the television screen all day can make us sore, stiff and underworked. So, what's the solution? Yoga, of course.

Yoga can help lengthen, strengthen, and stretch your muscles, thereby taking away most of your tension. Now, if you do not wish to spare a few minutes a day practicing yoga poses and don't mind paying huge money to masseur every day, you can feel to do so. But if you are a smart cookie like me, you will choose to yoga every day.

Lowers blood pressure

Coming back to the point where we spoke about how stress can cause our cortisol levels to rise, it can also increase our blood pressure levels. And I am sure all of you are aware how high dangerous high blood pressure levels can be for the body. But for those of you who need to hear the specifics, the impact of high blood pressure levels on our bodies include a risk of stroke, kidney damage, memory loss, heart attack and many others which you want to say away from.

High blood pressure, just like hypertension, is experienced when the blood that travels through our circulatory system exerts excessive pressure on the walls of our arteries. The reason why this happens can be various, including, stress, diet, disease, etc. Yoga can help eliminate stress-induced spike in blood pressure levels if practiced mindfully and repeatedly.

That's not to say that you have to stop your blood pressure medication and suddenly switch to yoga. However, if you continue to practice yoga, you will notice that your blood pressure will soon get back to normal.

Chapter 4: Seven Different Types of Meditation Practices

The process of meditation is deeply connected to yoga. While yoga involves focusing on your body and breathing, meditation makes you focus on your mind. Meditation is best practiced in silence, but you can also practice it while in the office, college, while working out or while you are on the go by simply focusing on your breath for a few seconds.

Meditation has gained a lot of popularity in the recent years as more and more people are looking to find a way to reduce their stress. In fact, there has been scientific evidence that proves that meditation can be a great tool for fighting chronic depression, chronic illnesses, chronic pain and even heart disease.

There are many different types of meditation practices. Here's a list of the most commonly used meditation techniques.

Mindfulness meditation

Mindfulness meditation is a process that keeps you fully aware of your thoughts. It helps you be present whenever different thoughts arise. Being mindful makes you aware of your thoughts, your actions, what we are doing, why we are doing it, and to control our emotional responses to our impulses. It makes you highly aware of your surroundings.

Mindful meditation can be performed just about anywhere. Like mentioned earlier, if you cannot sit in a quiet place, then you can do this meditation wherever you are. All you need to do is focus on your breath for as long as you can. It doesn't matter if you can't focus on more than 5 breaths, but if you do this frequently, you will start experiencing a sense of peace around you. Whenever you focus on your breath, your thoughts might start to overwhelm you, and you need to practice non-judgment to let them go.

Transcendental meditation

Transcendental meditation is an easy method that requires you to repeat a particular word or a phrase in a specific way. This technique is used in order to avoid distracting thoughts and promote a relaxed awareness. While performing this type of meditation, you need to sit in a comfortable position. You can sit on a chair, sofa or even on the floor. Just make sure that you are not leaning on anything. Now you need to close your eyes and repeat a mantra. What is mantra? A mantra is a sound or word used form the Vedic tradition for focusing.

Unlike other forms of meditation, which can be performed by anyone without any training, TM requires a 7-step course form a certified teacher. A certified transcendental teacher can guide you properly through the complete technique and explain its effect on human mind.

The idea behind TM is to allow you to get in a complete state of relaxed awareness where your only goal is to achieve mental peace.

Guided meditation

Guided meditation, which is also referred to as visualization technique or guided imagery, is one of the simplest forms of meditation. In this type of meditation, which is generally led by a teacher or a guide can take you through the steps of the entire meditation process by asking you to form mental pictures or events that you find relaxing.

Many guided meditation teachers will ask you to use your senses as much as possible such as sounds, texture, smell, etc. for triggering calm response in your space.

Vipassana meditation

Vipassana is an old Indian meditation practice. The term "Vipassana" refers to viewing things as they, without attaching any personal story to it. This type of meditation has been a part of Indian meditation practice over 2,500 years. In fact, the mindfulness meditation movement that took off in the United States is based on Vipassana meditation

The aim of Vipassana meditation is to transform your inner self through self-observation. This is accomplished by paying strict attention to all the physical sensations in the body in order to establish a strong connection between the body and the mind. The constant interconnectedness between the mind and the body leads to a balanced mind full of compassion and love. Typically, people who suffer from acute addictions such as alcohol, drugs, smoking or others take to Vipassana meditation.

Traditionally, Vipassana is a self-taught 10 day meditation course where the students are required to follow certain rules throughout their time in the Vipassana room. The rules include abstaining from intoxicants, any kind of sexual activity, stealing, telling lies, or killing of any species.

Loving kindness meditation (Metta Meditation)

Metta meditation, also known as the loving kindness meditation, is a meditation practice that teaches you to direct your well wishes towards everyone who comes in contact with you, including people on the street. People who practice the Metta meditation recite particular words or phrases that evoke warm hearted feeling within themselves and eventually in others around them. This practice is also commonly found in Vipassana as well as mindfulness meditation.

Loving kindness meditation is practiced by being seated in a relaxed and comfortable position. Now take a few full breaths and start repeating these words slowly, "May I be blessed. I may I be safe, May I be kind, May I be loving, May I be at peace."

Once you practice directing all the loving and kindness towards your own self, you can start imagining a close family member or even a friend who has been kind to you, and then repeat the above mantra again; except this time, replace the "I" with "you."

As you continue chanting the mantras, you can keep picturing a member of your family, your partner, friends, neighbors, people you bump into on a regular basis or even your pet. Several Vipassana practitioners encourage visualizing the images of people who we are currently struggling to deal with or have struggled in the past.

Lastly, you can end your meditation session using the universal Vipassana mantra, "May all beings everywhere be happy."

Chakra Meditation

Chakra is basically a Sanskrit term that means "wheel "and finds its roots in India. What are chakras? Chakras refer to the different centers of energy located in our body as well as the spiritual powers in them. There are seven different chakras. Every single chakra is rooted in a different part of your body and also has a corresponding color.

Chakra meditation consists of various relaxation techniques that focus on bringing about a balance as well as well-being to the chakras in your body. Experts claim that any kind of imbalance among the chakras is the reason why people suffer from emotional, mental and physical problems. Once these chakras are balanced, life is slowly brought back to normal, helping you taking better decisions, communicate effectively and feel all the emotions without suppressing them. Some of the techniques sue din chakra meditation included imagining every chakra in your body as well as its corresponding color. Don't worry if you don't know the colors of every chakra, your instructor will guide you through it.

Some people also prefer using crystals or incense sticks that are color coded for every single chakra for helping them focus through the meditation.

Chapter 5: Different Types of Yoga Poses and Stretches

Downward facing dog (Adho Mukha Svanasana)

- Start with your knees and hand, with your knees under the hips and hands stacked under the shoulders.
- Now spread both your hands as wide as you can and then press your thumb and index finger into the mat.
- Lift your tailbone slightly and press your butt a little up and back while drawing the hips towards the ceiling. Try straightening your legs as much as you can and press both your heels on the floor.
- Your head needs to rest between your arms, they should face your knees, and you should be lying flat on the back.
- Hold this position for a few seconds or up to 10 breaths.

Remember, that your focus here should be to keep your spine long- even if that means that you would need to bend your knees. This position could put a bit of pressure on your wrist. So, to avoid this, spread all your fingers, grab the mat using your fingertips and exert more weight on the pad where your first thumb and finger is and then insert them inside your palm.

Mountain pose/Tadasana

- Stand straight adjacent to a wall with your toes together and both the heels slightly apart.
- Spread your toes and spread your weight evenly between both feet. Here, you are required to engage your core muscles with your hips are tucked slightly while your tailbone if pointing towards the floor. Relax your arms and slowly roll them back down.

- Take a deep breath and lift your arms overhead while you press down into your feet. Alternatively, you can also choose to join your hands as if you are in prayer, by placing them in front of your chest – you can use any of these commonly used variations. If you are working with an instructor, it's possible that he or she may cue one specifically for you depending upon his style of training, and that's fine too.
- Now, while in this position, take long, slow and deep breaths through your nose.
- Hold this position for a few seconds or up to 10 breaths.

Try keeping your arms parallel to your ears. You can even slightly widen your arms if you need to.

Crescent Lunge/Utthita Ashwa Sanchalanasana

- You need to take a long step ahead with your right foot for starting with a staggered posture and keep your feet apart, about the length of the mat.
- Now, bend your right knee, keep your left leg in a straight posture and lift your heel from the floor. Start bending your right leg so that your thigh is placed parallel to the floor. Place your hips in the square position towards the front.
- Extend both your arms towards the ceiling. Try to stretch them up as you start pressing into the mat. At this point, try to feel the stretch in the hips fully.
- Hold this position for a few seconds or up to 10 breaths.
- Repeat the same on the other side.
- For moving into the low lunge position or Anjanayesana, all you need to do is drop your back knee onto the floor, keep the other leg extended long and your shin flat on the mat.

NOTE: It is vital to keep your spine long at all times. You can feel free to bend the back leg if it's helping your lift your torso while lengthening your back.

Warrior II / Virabhadrasana

- You need to take a long step forward with your right foot for starting with a staggered stance and keeping your feet about mat-length apart.
- Extend both your arms wide open, parallel to the floor.
- Bend your right knee to a near 90-degree angle, place your thigh parallel to the floor and keep the right leg straight.
- Start pointing your right toe forward while turning your left foot out towards the right hip in a way that it becomes perpendicular to the left foot.
- On the other hand, twist your torso a little towards the left so that your right hip faces towards the front and the left hip faces the back. Make sure that both your right arm as well as your head points forward while your left arm points towards the back.
- Hold this position for a few seconds or up to 10 breaths.

Note: Ensure that your right knee does not move past the ankle, and if it accidentally does, then try to reduce the depth of the lunge slightly.

Triangle/Trikonasana

- Start this pose in Warrior II
- Start straightening your front leg. Now, reach forward using your right hand towards the floor. Twist your torso slightly forward and start rotating it to open to the left side.
- Now, rotate both your arms to 6 and 12 o clock respectively. Place your right hand on the shin or on the

floor, is possible, and start extending the top arm fingers pointing towards the ceiling.

- Hold this position for a few seconds or up to 10 breaths.
- Repeat the same on the other side.

Note: Always keep your spine long. You can also use a block under your bottom hand for adding more stability to the pose.

Plank Pose/Kumbhakasana

- Begin on all fours. Place your knees under your hips, hands flat on the floor straight under your shoulders.
- Now try lifting your knees above the floor while extending both your legs out behind you. At this point, you should be on your hands and toes while your body forms a single long line.
- Place your palms flat on the floor, your hands arm-length apart, and your shoulders stacked above the wrist, and keep your core engaged. It's important to keep your spine and neck in a neutral position by facing down at the top of the mat.
- Hold this position for a few seconds or up to 10 breaths.

Note: At any given point of time if you feel that you straying away from the right form, stop and try again. Remember, posture is everything, especially when it comes to this pose.

Low Plank/Chaturanga Dandasana

- Again, start with the plank pose. Place your palms flat on the floor, your hands arm-length apart, and your shoulders stacked above the wrist, keep your core engaged and legs extended.
- Slowly start lowering down into a low plank pose by gently bending your elbows while you keep them tucked in towards the side of your body. The elbows should be tucked in a way that they form 90-degree angles.

- Now, hold this position for one single breath.
- Traditionally, this pose can be followed by the Upward-facing dog position.

The trick is not let your shoulders come any lower than your elbow-height. It's absolutely fine to do this move from your knees if you are unable to keep up with the conventional form. If you use your knees to perform this pose for a few days, you can slowly try performing it using your toes.

Upward-Facing Dog/Urdhva Mukha Svanasana

- Start with the low plank position by dropping your hips down on the floor while flipping your toes over in order to let the top of the feet touch the floor.
- Take a deep, full breath.
- Tighten your core by feeling every single muscle in the abdomen and straighten both your arms for pushing your chest up. Now, start pulling your shoulders back, squeeze the shoulder blades slightly and gently tilt your head facing the ceiling. This can help open up your chest. While you are doing this don't forget to keep breathing.

Note: At any point of time if you feel that the tension in the lower back is too much to handle, feel free to drop your knees. If it gets worse, you can completely skip this pose and try the High plank instead. For this, you have to observe how your body feels and switch the pose accordingly.

Tree/Vrikshasana

- Start this asana with a mountain pose by keeping both your toes together and heels apart.
- Now, bring the left foot towards the inner thigh of your right leg. Squeeze your foot as well as the inner thigh gently. The knee of the left leg should be turned out

whereas your left thigh should face downwards forming a 45-degree angle.

- Once you find your balance, you can simply lift your hands in a prayer position in front of the chest, or even place them overhead if it suits you.
- Your gaze needs to be focused on a certain point in front of you for helping you stay balanced. Do not close your eyes, keep them wide open but focus on an object in front of you.
- Hold this position for a few seconds or up to 10 breaths.
- Repeat the same on the other side.

Note: If you have any problem with balancing, you can try to place your left foot on your right shin instead of your thigh.

Dancers Pose/Natarajasana

- Start by standing tall with your feet together.
- Bend your right knee slightly while bringing your right foot towards the glutes. Grab tightly onto the inner arch of the right foot using your right hand and by slowly lifting the foot towards the ceiling.
- Start actively pressing down the floor using your entire left foot as you start opening the chest and pull the lifted up. Ensure to keep the chest lifted.
- Hold this position for a few seconds or up to 10 breaths.
- Repeat the same on the other side.

Note: Focus on keeping your hips at an even level. This will help lower your back in a comfortable position while avoiding overextension.

Half Pigeon Pose/Ardha Kapotasana

- From the downward facing dog position, start extending your right leg high while bringing your left leg underneath the body and place it right in front of you. AT the same time, ensure your shin is parallel to the top of the mat.

- Start extending your left leg behind you while resting the top of the foot straight on the floor.
- Keep your right foot flexed up. Try keeping your left hip as close to the mat as possible. In case it starts lifting off the floor, bring the right foot slightly closer to your body.
- Stay in this position for about three consecutive breaths. Now fold over while resting your head on the floor for about 10 breaths.
- Repeat the same on the other side.

Note: If you feel even the slightest bit of knee pain while trying to perform this pose, try the reclined figure four. In order to perform this pose, lie on the back while crossing your right foot over the left thigh while keeping the right foot flexed.

Seated Forward Fold/Pashchimottanasana

- Sit comfortably with your spine erect and both your legs extended in front of you. Now flex your feet a little. Sit tall with a straight back.
- Bend from your hips, keep your back flat and fold the upper body right over the lower body.
- If possible, grab tightly on the outside of both feet, or your shin or ankles.
- Start releasing your neck while letting the head hang heavy.
- Hold this position for a few seconds or up to 10 breaths.
- Repeat the same on the other side.

Note: You can absolutely bend your knees if you have to until you can tip the pelvis forward and your back lengthens.

Conclusion

I wish to thank you once again for purchasing this book.

Yoga has changed my life in a magical way that cannot be translated into words. I want all my readers to make yoga a part of their life, and not just as a form of exercise or a tool to achieve peace.

When you embrace yogic practice as a way of life, your life will start changing in ways you cannot imagine. You will experience moments of euphoria without being high on any external drug. I consider this guide as an opportunity to educate my readers about all that I have known and experienced about yoga.

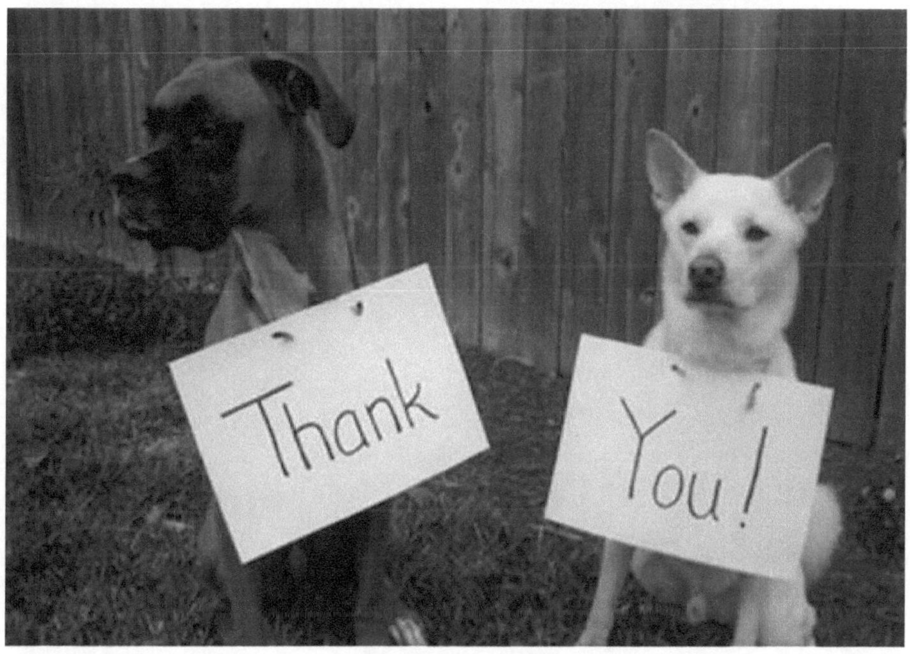

Finally, if you enjoyed this book and found it useful, then I'd like to ask you for a favor, would you be kind enough to leave a review for this book on Amazon? It'd be greatly appreciated! ***Please do it now!!***, it will take just a few minutes of your time...otherwise you might get so busy you'll forget.

Click here OR TYPE (https://amzn.to/2U4PMhH) for review

Thank you and good luck!